POSITIVE VOICES

FACE TO FACE WITH HIV/AIDS

POSITIVE VOICES

FACE TO FACE WITH HIV/AIDS

Edited by

Dr. Subhash Hira   Dr. Manisha Sen   Rajendar Menen

SAṀSKṚITI

ARCON

SAṀSKṚITI
C-9020 Vasant Kunj, New Delhi-110070
in collaboration with
Aids Research and Control Centre (ARCON)
Skin & STD Building
Sir J. J. Hospital, Mumbai-400008

First Published 1999
Second impression 2000

 The scientific information provided in this book is meant for training and education of health-care workers. All names, characters and identities have been changed to protect HIV-positive individuals. Any resemblance of name and identity with an individual, living or dead, is coincidental. The contents do not reflect the policy or opinion of the Government of Maharashtra, the University of Texas-Houston, AIDS Research & Control Centre, Mumbai, or MGM Medical College, Navi Mumbai.

ISBN 81-87374-05-5

Printed at Reprographics India, New Delhi.
Published by M. Sengupta for Saṁskṛiti, New Delhi, in association with Arcon-Mumbai.

ABOUT THE EDITORS

Dr. Subhash Hira is Professor of Infectious Diseases at the University of Texas-Houston on assignment to the Government of Maharashtra as the Director of the ARCON Centre, Mumbai. A physician-specialist, he has worked with the HIV/AIDS epidemic in Africa, America and India. He has served as technical advisor to NACO and the World Bank.

Dr. Manisha Sen is a Clinical Psychologist. Professor and Head of the University Department of Applied Psychology, University of Mumbai, she is also a Senate Member of the University of Mumbai and a Consultant to UNAIDS. She is an expert on the training of counsellors for HIV/AIDS.

Rajendar Menen is the Executive Editor of *AIDS Update*, Mumbai. Recipient of the first Lilian Khare award, he has written over two thousand articles is more than thirty journals in five countries. He has also authored over a hundred articles on AIDS and related issues and been involved in more than ten television documentaries on the subject. He has lecutred in Europe, been a consultant to the UNFPA and freelanced for the BBC.

ACKNOWLEDGEMENT

The editors acknowledge the contributions of Ms Sunita Ramkumar, Counselling Psychologist and Sonal Shinde, Social Psychologist, the technical assistance of Dr. Clemente Fernandes and the clinical unit of the ARCON Centre and the staff of the Sir J.J. Hospital, Mumbai, and the MGM Hospital, Kamothe.

OTHER TITLES OF INTEREST

SEXUALITY AND HIV/AIDS

The book deals with issues of sexuality of Persons Living With HIV/AIDS (PLWHA) and documents in-depth life experiences of PLWHA, their self-expression and biases towards sexuality. The book documents the complex and diverse maze of lifetime sexual partners and carries illustrated the "sexual tree" of individuals. These individuals represent unseleted faces within the Indian Society. Each of the 30-odd case studies end with important observations provided by editors and deal with issues of sexual behaviour and risk taking. This book is tailored towards the need of health-care workers who deal with PLWHA on a regular basis. It is to be the only resource material for training of HIV/AIDS counsellors and clinicians. Authors believe that this book, first of its kind in India, will have a wider impact on the Indian society in terms of modification of sexual behaviour towards safer sex.

HANDBOOK OF CLINICAL MANAGEMENT OF HIV/AIDS

This comprehensive handbook on HIV/AIDS covers commonly encountered HIV-related illnesses, opportunistic infections, and related malignancies. With expanding base of HIV/AIDS epidemic in India, there is an urgent need for decentralised care services at the district level. Hence, the book written in simple language is accompanied with ample illustrations (clinical slides, radiographs, microscopic slides, tables and flowcharts) to meet needs of health-care workers at the district level. This will fulfill the need for updated information in the ever-changing field of HIV/AIDS. Authors of this book are committed to decentralised clinical case management of HIV/AIDS in public and private care institutions. This should help decongest tertiary level hospitals in India.

CONTENTS

FOREWORD

HIV is an epidemic that has reached alarming proportions globally. In India this rapid spread is mainly because issues related to sexuality are always swept under the carpet. The clinical aspect of the disease is fairly well managed. However, there is a major lacuna in the management of the psycho-social issues concerning people living with AIDS.

For an HIV-positive individual, a doctor can only help in treating his or her opportunistic infections. It is the counsellor who provides the continuing support which is very crucial considering the fact that those who test HIV-positive are discriminated against by society. The extensive discrimination is mainly due to ignorance about the disease and the non-availability of a cure.

This book aims at capturing the wide spectrum of psycho-social concerns of people living with AIDS, exploring the dynamics of the process of counselling, and to enable counsellors who are new to this field to prepare themselves adequately. For a good counsellor it is essential to keep abreast of recent developments in the field of HIV/AIDS. This book can be used as a reference guide by health care workers as it includes most of the critical psycho-social problems faced by people living with AIDS.

I understand that this book documents true case histories as narrated by the clients to the counsellors.

All the cases included in this book are of patients regularly following up at the ARCON Centre at Grant Medical

College and Sir J. J. Hospital in Mumbai. Counselling is an ongoing process. Most clients came from a variety of social backgrounds and had divergent psycho-social concerns. After repeated counselling sessions, most of them saw a ray of hope and developed a desire to lead a healthy life. Many of the case studies also depict the unnecessary suffering and discrimination that a client faces due to his or her HIV-positive status.

I hope that these case studies will give the right orientation to AIDS health-care workers to empathise with HIV-positive individuals in a more meaningful manner. I wish this publication all success.

Thomas C. Benjamin, IAS

Secretary, Medical Education & Drugs Department

Government of Maharashtra

Chairperson, ARCON Advisory Committee

INSIGHT

We have put together case studies in the book highlighting various psychological issues and concerns of people living with HIV/AIDS. Through this endeavour, we have taken an opportunity to share our experiences and our growth as counsellors working in the field of HIV/AIDS.

Our background and training in psychology had provided us with a framework that was essential for working in a service oriented profession. But HIV/AIDS counselling was just one of the many topics that we covered in our academic life.

However, it was through our practical experience of working in this field at the ARCON Centre at the Sir J. J. Hospital that we enriched our knowledge and gained a deeper insight into the various aspects of HIV/AIDS counselling. At the outset itself, the uniqueness of the chronic illnesses associated with HIV/AIDS was apparent to us as compared to other life-threatening illnesses. The care and management of persons with HIV/AIDS is a complex process which requires a multidisciplinary team comprising physicians, counsellors, nurses, laboratory technologists, and the family of the client. Understanding this complex process and developing collaborations at all levels which then work together to provide proper care of persons with HIV/AIDS is a marathon. We are glad to have been participants in this marathon.

At the outset, anxiety seems to be the predominant emotion most persons face before the HIV-test, during the waiting period for the result and when the report is being disclosed; more so if the report reveals an HIV-positive status. However, the other accompanying or precipitating emotions/

reactions differ based on the personality and the situation of the individual. These include fear, denial, guilt, anger, frustration, resignation, acceptance and even indifference.

There were other aspects besides individual reactions that widened the focus of counselling. Issues related to sexuality, partner counselling and testing, marriage, pregnancy, children, social stigma, discrimination, support needs, employment, disease progression and death.

During the process of HIV/AIDS counselling, we had to reaffirm the principles and techniques learnt during our academic life: principles such as empathy, acceptance, unconditional positive regard and non-judgemental attitude towards all our clients. These principles are the building blocks of the process of counselling through which a rapport was established with clients to empower them to help themselves.

In our capacity as HIV/AIDS counsellors we realised the significance and the practical application of these techniques and their influence on the process of counselling resulting in a growth-oriented relationship with the client.

This process of growth helped us become more introspective, become more aware of our limitations and strengths, our hidden biases and prejudices and helped us find ways of overcoming them.

We discovered that we were faced with numerous challenges in the process of HIV/AIDS counselling. These included:

* Providing support and encouragement to clients despite knowing that there is no cure as yet in sight;

* Motivating non-compliant clients to develop self-reliance;

* Ascertaining if the client is unwilling to discuss certain issues and not needle him/her for further information;

* Initiating discussions on sexuality and contraception despite cultural inhibitions, the lack of a proper vocabulary for sexuality and gender biases;

* Developing sensitivity to understand the various socio-economic, cultural and financial pressures on the client who is already burdened with the diagnosis of an incurable infection;

* Maintaining a difficult balance between objectivity and the need to empathise; and

* Developing mechanisms to counter fatigue, feelings of monotony, repetition and eventual burn-out.

While we have successfully faced these challenges and difficulties during counselling, we have also gained a lot from our experiences. It has been an extremely enriching and enlightening process. We have grown both professionally and personally. We have observed the crucial role played by family, friends and society in times of need. We have also seen how families resolve their differences to provide care and support to their sick ones. The most significant lesson learnt is that the bonding between individuals is much stronger than what is apparent. Most of our clients have the will to live.

We have gained strength from the positive people we have worked with and this strength helps us to give of our best. This strength also furthers our resolve to continue providing quality care.

Sunita Ramkumar, M.A. (Psychology)

Sonal Shinde, M.A.(Psychology)

CASE 1

SINGLE MALE: SELF-DESTRUCTIVE BEHAVIOUR

MURGESH is a thirty-year-old, unmarried hawker who sells odds and ends at a tiny stall in the central business district of south Mumbai. He has studied till the eighth standard in English and revealed a strange life story.

Murgesh's father died while he was in the seventh standard and his mother married the family driver with whom she was having a protracted affair. In disgust, he left his home in the western suburbs of Mumbai. He was a child then without any support systems. But he preferred the mean streets of Mumbai for shelter and a livelihood. This was home now. He had decided never to look back.

Emaciated, dirty, unkempt and sick looking, Murgesh was initially very defensive when he came to the ARCON Centre at the Sir J. J. Hospital for medical attention and counselling. He expected to be reprimanded for not having collected his HIV report earlier. He had come exactly a year after his HIV test and pre-test counselling. He appeared strong-willed and wanted to live life on his own terms. He spoke fluent English and seemed nonchalant about his HIV-positive status.

Living on the streets of Mumbai, Murgesh had innumerable and unusual experiences. But despite the new twists and turns in his life, he loved talking about his family. His father, he said, was a brilliant man. He had his own business and was doing well in life. They also shared a very good rapport. He was devastated when his father expired. He had a drinking problem but what really killed him, according to Murgesh, was his mother's affair with their driver.

Murgesh was not mature enough at that time to understand the implications of his mother's behaviour. He blamed her for his father's death. When he realised that the driver would now take his father's place in the house, he couldn't take it any longer. He packed his bags and left home. He was only fourteen years old then. But he was ambitious and determined to do well in life. He wanted to take care of his mother and divorced sister and "rescue" them from the clutches of "that man".

On the streets his money ran out in no time. He began eating at roadside stalls and sleeping at railway platforms and in abandoned trains in the yard. During the last fifteen years his circle of acquaintances included eunuchs, petty thieves, ragpickers, commercial sex workers, mafia dons, policemen and other runaways. He had been chased by the law and had been hurt in street brawls. He had also picked up a variety of odd jobs and had travelled the length and breadth of the country by train. He felt that he had seen life in its ugliest forms. At thirty, he was a veteran. Streetsmart, his instincts were honed like an animal in the wild, fully capable of looking after himself in the urban jungle.

When Murgesh left home he had hoped to make sufficient money to educate himself. But the harsh realities of the road had other ideas. He had to stretch his wits to survive. Success in the conventional sense eluded him. Society considered him a deviant, the law inflicted pain whenever it wound its long tentacles around him and his family considered him a black sheep. He felt frustrated and dejected.

While in Indore during his many wanderings, Murgesh met another runaway and they became good friends. Like him, this new friend also belonged to a good family but had run away from home and had vowed never to return. Murgesh also met his friend's sister and in due course fell in love with her. He decided to marry her and broached the subject with his friend who had by then settled his differences with his family and was preparing to go back to them.

When he heard Murgesh's proposal he was furious. He didn't want his sister to marry a good-for-nothing street urchin. He threatened Murgesh with serious harm if he kept with his intentions and asked him to leave Indore immediately. This friend was well connected, and Murgesh had no choice. Disillusioned, hurt and angry, he began having sex indiscriminately on the rebound. He didn't take recourse in alcohol or drugs, but began sleeping with any woman he met. He was eighteen years old then. There were many like him living on the streets. It was easy. Of course, condoms were never used.

Soon, Murgesh developed Sexually Transmitted Diseases (STDs) and tuberculosis. He kept falling sick. He was hospitalised for malaria. Though not formally informed, he was aware of HIV/AIDS. He came to the ARCON Centre for a test on his own initiative but returned for the report only a year later. Immediately after the test, he was hospitalised. Quite certain he was HIV-positive, he decided there was little point in getting the report. But he began falling ill more frequently as the months passed and decided to get proper medical attention.

When Murgesh came for counselling, the counsellor had to first deal with his defensive stance. The counsellor assured him that she was not going to reprimand him. Instead, she tried to understand his reasons for not coming to collect his HIV test report for a year. This helped greatly and resulted in Murgesh simply opening up and narrating his entire life story. It was quite apparent from listening to him that he carried a load of negative emotions from the past and all that luggage was troubling him. Through the process of counselling, he would have to get in touch with those feelings, acknowledge them and analyse them rationally and productively.

The counsellor emphasised the importance of focusing on the present and future rather than on the past. Murgesh was encouraged to consider his priorities (whether to stay on his own or go back to his family who had repeatedly approached him) vis-à-vis his current HIV status.

After repeated counselling, Murgesh realised the need to take care of himself. He is now being treated for opportunistic infections and has even begun thinking about approaching his mother, burying the past and starting anew.

OBSERVATIONS

* Fragile emotional state arising out of unfavourable home environment is reflected. Knowledge of the mother's illicit

relationship with the driver resulted in feelings of disgust and resentment.

* Evidence of self-destructive behaviour of leaving home and taking to the streets is a presentation of maladaptive coping mechanisms used to meet life stressors.

* The client's decision to renew his relationship with his mother indicates the realisation of the need to connect with the family as a support system.

* The drop-out rate among clients returning for their HIV test results at the ARCON Centre is two per cent. The instances of drop-outs could be due to denial on the part of the client, casual attitude with regard to health issues, migration out of Mumbai or death.

* Vulnerability of street children in terms of compromises made in life in areas like food, shelter, health, sex education, safety, security and human values.

* Street children should be priority individuals for targeted intervention.

* There is the need to popularise family counselling as a preventive strategy.

CASE 2

SINGLE MALE: DISCRIMINATION AND LACK OF SUPPORT

SADANAND, a forty-year-old bachelor, worked as a domestic help in the house of a government official in Byculla in central Mumbai. He came to Mumbai from Vijayawada twenty-four years ago. His parents died when he was three years old and he began living with his uncle and aunt. But he ran away from home as he was being ill-treated by them. He had, by then, studied till the eighth standard in the English medium.

In 1973 Sadanand met with a road accident. He was hospitalised. His jaw bone was completely smashed and he was fitted with artificial teeth. His recovery process was long and protracted. In hospital he was transfused four units of blood but he was lucky, in a way, because the owner of the vehicle which hit him paid for his hospitalisation and even employed him in his factory.

Sadanand was meticulously dressed when he came for the counselling session. He said he preferred white clothes because it symbolised purity. He was clean-shaven and had worn a couple of chains and rings. He had a sharp nasal tone and gestured a lot. He also had evident feminine mannerisms. He was very talkative and said his friends called him a livewire. He said he wanted to spread happiness in life and believed that God would punish those who troubled him. He also loved painting and tried his hand at fashion designing and modelling with little success.

In his present job, Sadanand was entrusted with all the household chores. He had no fixed salary but he got a place to stay, food to eat, occasional pocket money and a lot of love from his adopted family.

The lady of the house was a school teacher, two daughters were doctors and the son a computer engineer. Sadanand was very fond of the family and had no complaints. In turn, he said, they trusted him with their lives.

In January 1996 Sadanand had a severe bout of jaundice. The elder daughter asked him to undergo a thorough medical check-up. He tested HIV-positive. All of a sudden, according to him, the love and care the family had for him vanished. He was then discouraged from entering the kitchen, wasn't allowed to meet anybody, and when a grand daughter was born was asked to keep away from her. He was told that his life was over and he must not spoil anybody else's.

Sadanand was shattered by this sudden turnaround in the behaviour of his adopted family. His employer had promised to set him up in a private business with some seed money but had now gone back on his promise. He was also constantly told that he had engaged in immoral acts and God was punishing him for it. Sadanand was now completely isolated.

The counsellor suggested that he discuss with the family

issues like discrimination, his dues for the work done etc. This would involve identifying a member of the family to whom he could present his case in a cool and composed manner. If that didn't work, he could approach any voluntary organisation which provided legal help to HIV-positive patients.

But Sadanand was scared. He believed his adopted family would harm him if he went to court. He was in a very precarious position. He insisted that he had never had drugs or any sexual exposure. The virus, he said, was passed on to him during the blood transfusion twenty-five years ago!

OBSERVATIONS

* Client may have had negative perceptions of his relatives' behaviour towards him during his childhood. This led to his running away from home.

* Informal adoption of the client could mean that there is no formal relationship between the employer and the employee.

* Sexual orientation of the client appears ambiguous and therefore it is difficult to ascertain the route of HIV transmission.

* Ostracism of an HIV-positive person by a doctor who is expected to be a role model for the community.

* Judgemental attitude of the adopted family seems to have instilled feelings of worthlessness, guilt and isolation.

* Need for popularising the role of organisations providing supportive services like psychological, legal, social and financial aid.

CASE 3

COMMERCIAL SEX WORKER: CONFLICTING EMOTIONS

ANITA, a twenty-one-year-old commercial sex worker, was referred to the ARCON Centre for supportive counselling. She had tested HIV-positive and the purpose of the counselling session was to provide her options outside the flesh trade. She had told the counsellor at the rehabilitation centre where she was temporarily housed that she wanted to return to her profession as a commercial sex worker as soon as possible. The brothel was her only home now. The outside world, she said, was an alien place.

When Anita arrived at the ARCON Centre she was wearing the rehabilitation centre's uniform. Tall, dark and very attractive, she also appeared determined and strong-willed.

Her story translated into English from colloquial Hindi:

"I am from a small village in Andhra Pradesh. I was brought to Mumbai by my uncle. I wanted to become a professional singer and he told me and my family that Mumbai was the city to launch my career. He promised me a job and talked to my parents about it. My parents didn't mind. They are very poor and required money. A monthly contribution from me was necessary for their upkeep.

"I was only fourteen years old when I came to Mumbai. It was the first time that I was getting away from my little village. The bus and train journeys and the big city were all new to me. I also knew no one in Mumbai. My uncle was the only support. But his behaviour changed dramatically as soon as we left home. When we reached Mumbai he sold me off to a brothel.

"The first few months were terrible. I was not allowed to go out or even talk to anybody. Many men were sent to my room. I didn't understand all this in the beginning. It was much later that it sank into me that I was part of a brothel and would have to sleep with different men for a livelihood. I was now a member of the world's oldest profession.

"Now I can't even go back home. My roots are cut. My uncle has told my parents that I am a prostitute. Of course, he didn't tell them that he was responsible for selling me to a brothel. This is my world now and I have to live with it.

"I am told I have the AIDS virus. I don't know how long I have had it or who infected me. We have so many customers that it is difficult to know. How can I know who has given me all these painful sores? But what pains me even more is the insensitivity of all the social workers who don't consider our feelings. They blame prostitutes for all the diseases in the city. I was not born a prostitute nor was I born with AIDS. Society gave it to me. How can I be blamed?

"When I was being treated for my sores I refused to take any customers. When my uncle knew of my ill health he stopped coming to see me. He stays close by and used to come regularly for money. Luckily that has stopped. Now only a part of my earnings will be given to the *gharwali*. I can keep the other part.

"There is one customer who comes to me regularly. My uncle used to restrict him from meeting me. Now I can meet him whenever I want to. I am very fond of him, maybe I am in love with him. That is another reason I want to leave the rehabilitation centre and go back to the brothel. Also, there is nothing for me to do at the centre. I am told by all the doctors that I may not live long. If that customer knows about my illness he may want to leave me too. Then I will have nothing left in life. So it is better that I go back to my business and earn some money fast so that I can live the rest of my life in comfort.

"I know I will be infecting my customers if I continue working in the brothel. But they deserve to be infected. But I wouldn't want their innocent wives and children to be infected for no fault of theirs. From now on I will insist on a condom. If a customer refuses, I won't take him on.

"It is very difficult for me to leave the profession. I earn a lot as a prostitute. The only alternative would be to work as a maidservant. But who will give me work? Anyway, I don't want to do that job. I have been in the brothel for many years now. I know all the other girls well. We are like a family. We help each other in pain and in sorrow. I feel secure there. I have friendship, food, clothes, a roof over my head and the customer I like very much. I will feel lost in the outside world. No, I can't leave the brothel and go anywhere else.

"But let me tell you something which will startle you. I am happy to get this disease. The doctors say it will never leave me. It will be the only thing that will remain faithful to me.

"I have lost everything, every single thing has been taken away from me. I have nothing. But now nobody can take this disease away from me.

"I know I am a prostitute. I live in a brothel and service many men. It is very easy to judge me and others who work with me. It is easy to blame us for everything that is wrong in society. But don't you see that somewhere society has failed in protecting a young girl and her family? There are hundreds of thousands of young and innocent girls who are forced into prostitution. These unfortunate circumstances are created by society. You would have done the same thing if you were in my place!"

The counsellors realised that Anita had a lot of anger against herself and society and so provided her the opportunity to ventilate her feelings. It was suggested that she direct her energies to options available and set goals accordingly.

OBSERVATIONS

* Prostitution is a significant social issue.

* The client appears to have experienced feelings of hopelessness and frustration.

* Conflicting emotions like revenge and empathy were present in the client. Counselling needs to be directed towards helping the client deal with them.

* There is a need for health care professionals to be non-judgemental and sensitive.

* It is necessary for health care professionals to adopt a

cautious approach while referring to HIV as an infection and AIDS as the terminal stage disease.

* Counsellor needs to work with the client to instil hope.

* The client needs to be prepared for the consequences of her dependence on a partner.

CASE 4

HOMOSEXUAL ORIENTATION: PSYCHOSOCIAL THREATS

ANAND Sarkar is thirty-six years old with a homosexual orientation. He is tall, slim and dark with curly hair. He has a soft voice, is always well dressed and his gestures and mannerisms betray a touch of femininity. Hailing from a middle-class family, he is a qualified accountant. His father, a government employee, passed away recently. He has a mother and three sisters who are married. The family resides in a one-room apartment in the western suburbs of Mumbai.

Right from childhood, Anand shunned familial obligations and lived life on his own terms without compromises or concessions to others. All this had distanced him from the family. Matters turned worse when he tested HIV-positive. The family was convinced they were right in considering him a deviant. Only one sister seemed to empathise with his plight. For the rest of the family he was a no-gooder who only contributed a lot of anger and disappointment to their lives.

They tolerated him at home but when he expressed a desire to leave and stay on his own there was no opposition whatsoever. They were probably glad he had finally decided to pack up and fend for himself.

The youngest of four children in a conservative, middle-class family, Anand grew up in the shadow of his three sisters. He frequently admitted at counselling sessions that his feminine mannerisms and thought processes were probably because of the influence of his sisters.

Anand's childhood wasn't a comfortable one. He was teased about his looks. His dark complexion and curly hair met with snide comments. All this lowered his self-esteem and exaggerated his insecurities.

In the tenth standard Anand had a sexual relationship with a male relative. He seemed to have enjoyed it. He started seeking out more encounters of the kind and also began to believe he was homosexual.

The trend continued in college. Anand realised he was different from the other boys. He wasn't attracted to girls. Instead, he felt intimidated and threatened by them. He was quite clearly uncomfortable in their presence. On the other hand, he became increasingly attracted to well dressed and good looking boys. His adolescent phase was turbulent. The ambiguity regarding his sexuality was tearing him apart. Confusion and torment were destroying him. He had nobody to reach out to, to share the distress that had seized his soul.

After college, Anand decided to become an accountant. He took seven years to complete the course. He frequently got distracted, lacked motivation, changed his plans often and generally moved along without purpose.

One day he went to a public toilet at a Mumbai railway station and witnessed scenes of blatant homosexual activity. His curiosity and interest were aroused. He started visiting all the toilets at various stations. This station hopping became a habit which kept him occupied till late at night. This met with the disapproval of his family, but Anand had long since stopped caring. It was during this period of his life that he came into contact with *Hijras* or eunuchs, and the seeds of a long association with them were sown.

Anand found work in a government organisation but it offered him no job satisfaction. He began to bunk work and spend the time in homosexual activities. His father resented every move of his and finally when the differences between them grew irreparable, Anand left the job for another city. With no one to check him now, this move was, in hindsight, a costly mistake.

Anand now began hanging around public places like parks and toilets soliciting clients. He balanced his escapades with his new job. But that was a tough act. He soon lost the job, was penniless and returned to home in Mumbai.

Back in Mumbai, Anand returned to his old habits. He started frequenting public toilets again. One day he was introduced to a powerful *Hijra* who was a sort of gangleader and engaged in a number of nefarious activities. As the days passed into weeks, Anand got to know the *Hijra* better and decided to move in with him into his small room in Goregaon in suburban Mumbai. Directionless, with no family or friend to tell him any better, Anand's life lurched from crisis to crisis.

Encouraged by the *Hijra*, Anand decided to earn quick money. He started hanging out at railway stations late at night. Invariably, he would be approached and picked up. Anand now became a male prostitute. He had no job, was living with the *Hijra,* had picked up the nuances of the trade and was making a living by offering his body to other men.

All this had its flip side. Anand fell prey to sexually transmitted diseases and his anal region was ruptured. When the *Hijra* realised that Anand was making a decent living, he demanded a slice of the cake. The slice started increasing in size. Unable to meet the *Hijra's* demands, Anand packed his bags and returned home yet again.

His parents didn't welcome him with open arms but they didn't shut the door on him either. But after Anand's stint with the *Hijra* and his exposure to the underbelly of homosexual activity in Mumbai, he had changed from deep within. The crack between him and his parents had widened further. He was now a complete stranger to them. To make matters worse, his suitcase was full of women's clothes. They had become his workclothes along with the elaborate make-up and the finery that contributed to the adornment of a beautiful woman. Anand had started cross-dressing after he met the *Hijras.* His conservative, middle-class parents were shocked beyond belief.

Meanwhile, he met another *Hijra* and went to live with him. When he tired of it, he returned home. By now Anand started falling sick regularly with a variety of infections. He also tested HIV-positive.

He wrote to his parents a long confessional letter detailing every misfortune. They sought expert medical advice. Not long after, his father died. Now Anand stays with his mother who is not very keen to have him at home. She is unable to nurse him during his frequent bouts of illness and also unable to fathom the medical attention required by an HIV-positive person.

Anand's main problem was one of acceptance; initially for his sexual orientation and now for his HIV-positive status. The counselling sessions were aimed at providing a non-judgemental atmosphere to fulfil the client's need to be accepted and understood. The client was encouraged to set goals for himself. It was suggested that he desist from high-risk behaviour and become part of a support group of positive persons.

Anand is now occupied with meetings and seminars about HIV/AIDS and getting as much information as he can about treatment options. He is following up for counselling at regular intervals. He is also a regular support group member.

OBSERVATIONS

* It is important for counsellors to understand that clients have different sexual orientations and to accept them as they are.

* The case reflects lack of support from the family due to non-acceptance of the client's sexual orientation.

* Issue of transvestism needs to be recognised.

* Training is necessary for family members of HIV-positive persons for home based care.

* The importance of encouraging the clients to form self-help groups is highlighted.

* Importance of follow-up and ongoing supportive counselling is evident in this case.

CASE 5

MARRIED COUPLE: STRESSORS OF URBAN MIDDLE-CLASS

THIS is the story of a couple who have been married for over a year. Shrikant is forty years old and works as a bus conductor. He had recurring bouts of fever, diarrhoea and sexually transmitted diseases. His family doctor advised him to get an HIV test done and he tested positive. Twenty-nine year-old Rachna, his wife, was also asked to undergo a test. Tall, thin, soft-spoken and reserved, Rachna also tested positive.

They were an economically disadvantaged couple. Shrikant was Rachna's sole support. She had five sisters and a brother but when she was only three years old she was adopted by her maternal uncle who had lost his wife. Living away from her siblings, she was unable to build a bond with them. While still at school, her uncle remarried and her step-aunt began ill-treating her. So Rachna returned to her parents' home. Though her parents weren't unkind, Rachna had by now lost all sense of belonging. She had lived away for too long. She felt unloved, insecure and unable to really communicate with anybody.

Rachna married Shrikant and moved into his house.The first three months were fine but after that her in-laws began harassing her. They began finding fault with everything she did and made her life miserable. Shrikant's loyalty was also divided between his wife and his family.

Shrikant explained that his father was the head of the family and made all the decisions which were followed without question. After his retirement, Shrikant took it upon himself to run the family which comprised his parents, two brothers and a sister. The going was tough. He had to do a number of odd jobs to make ends meet and even make personal sacrifices like postponing his marriage. After his father's death, the responsibilities increased. Somehow, Shrikant managed to fulfil his obligations but instead of gratitude and respect all he got from his siblings in return was resentment. These pressures, he says, drove him to commercial sex workers before marriage.

All this tension in the narrow confines of their tiny suburban apartment grew unbearable for the couple. Shrikant sometimes vented his anger on Rachna in front of the others. This seemed to hurt her the most and she used to get very depressed. She even contemplated suicide.

The pressure on the couple took a further twist. The family wanted them to have a child. Shrikant and Rachna also yearned for an offspring but were aware of the consequences. They didn't have the money or the space to bring another human being into the world. They were also HIV-positive which had been kept a secret from the others.

Since Shrikant and Rachna always came together to the ARCON Centre, they were often counselled together. In the beginning, it was invariably Shrikant who spoke and dominated the conversation. Rachna sat quietly, in a subdued manner. But often she conveyed through her non-verbal gestures that she did not quite agree to everything that her husband said. Hoping that she might open up better in the absence of her husband, Rachna was separately counselled. It was found that she was experiencing a lot of pain (especially in her relationship with her husband) which was taking precedence over the HIV-positive status.

Thus, it was necessary for the counsellor to tackle various personal issues such as the couple's relationship with the family and even the relationship between themselves. During the counselling, after a little probing, Shrikant admitted that the anger experienced by his siblings was not totally misplaced. His bossy attitude towards them, he felt, could have contributed to the resentment.

The counselling process was aimed at helping Rachna and Shrikant communicate better. It was intended to enable the couple to realise the importance of mutual support which would give them the strength and courage to cope better with circumstances.

The couple came for a follow-up visit soon after December1, World AIDS Day. The media hype which associated HIV with death had precipitated great emotional turmoil in their lives. This clearly indicated the need for more supportive, follow-up counselling sessions for the couple.

OBSERVATIONS

* Psychosocial pressures of do's and don'ts on a young couple from a middle-class family are evident; especially when they are already stressed with an incurable disease.

* Psychological trauma of the client during her childhood

seemed to have resulted in insecurities, non-assertiveness and lack of self-esteem which affected her interpersonal relationships as an adult.

* Inaccurate and flamboyant AIDS messages can have disastrous consequences.

* Need for timely identification of psychological crises such as suicidal tendencies, and the necessity of providing crisis counselling have to be addressed.

* Counselling to improve interpersonal communication between the couple seems to be imperative.

* Developing decision making skills to help deal with social pressures is another goal of counselling in this case.

■ CASE 6 ■

MARRIED COUPLE: ACCEPTANCE OF HIV-POSITIVE STATUS

JOHN and Esther were sent to the ARCON Centre for clinical management of HIV. Esther had tested HIV-positive during an antenatal clinic screening. She had subsequently delivered a baby boy. Later, John had also tested HIV-positive at a private laboratory in Mumbai city.

Twenty-six years old, John has been married for a year-and-a-half. He worked as a contract worker and had no steady income. Slightly built and educated till the ninth standard, he had very little knowledge of HIV/AIDS apart from the sexual mode of transmission. He was receptive to whatever the counsellor said. John pointed out that he had no history of sexual exposure and was quite surprised by the report although his HIV-positive status was confirmed at the ARCON Centre. He presented no psychological problems and wondered how he could have been infected.

A twenty-three year-old housewife who had also studied till the ninth standard, Esther asked many relevant questions about HIV. She gave no history of any high-risk behaviour. Her only worry was her son's health and if the infection would be passed on to him.

The couple lived in a joint family. John's parents, his younger brother and a younger sister stayed with them. His father worked in a shop, his brother worked as a technician and his sister worked in a plastic goods manufacturing company. The couple's HIV status was known to everybody at home.

At the post-test counselling session, John wanted to know if a woman could transmit HIV to a man. When the counsellor said that was possible, John seemed pleased. He said his in-laws were accusing him of being unfaithful and infecting their daughter. They had even asked him to send their daughter back. Esther, however, wanted to remain with John but had not succeeded in convincing her parents.

John pointed out that the next time his in-laws accused him of infecting their daughter, he would tell them it was the other way around and that he was the one who had been betrayed. The counsellor asked him whether he really felt betrayed by his wife. He said he didn't and that he would only use this information as ammunition against his in-laws. The counsellor asked him if Esther could be called in and if all of them could sit together and talk. He agreed and Esther joined the counselling session.

They sat face to face and began discussing the issue threadbare. The counsellor was present only as a facilitator and did not intervene until they wanted her to. Esther and John discussed their feelings for each other and decided to stick together through the worst of times. After the counselling sessions, John decided that there was no point in looking for scapegoats. What had happened had happened!

Esther had remained silent through all the earlier counselling sessions. She finally said that she was keen on putting the past behind her and staying on with her husband. They had to fight the problem together. Both of them also decided to talk to their families openly. Accusations and counter accusations, they felt, were leading them nowhere.

In this case, the counsellor's role was to prepare the ground for opening channels of communication between the couple.

OBSERVATIONS

* Issues emerging out of 'unconsented' HIV testing in an ante-natal clinic are highlighted in this case.

* The burden on John of being blamed for betraying Esther seemed to have taken precedence over being HIV-positive.

* Ownership of responsibility of HIV transmission lies with both partners in this case and is not necessarily male driven.

* Couple counselling helped to facilitate acceptance of HIV-positive status and its associated psychological implications such as stigma and blame.

* Family counselling involving Esther's parents can help shift focus from the past to the present and the future.

* There was the realisation of the importance of mutual support and encouragement in facing HIV illness and its consequences.

CASE 7

FAMILY REACTIONS: CONCEPT OF PSYCHOSOCIAL COUNSELLING

TWENTY-EIGHT year-old Amrik Singh completed his secondary school examinations and followed it up with a technical course which he didn't complete. His family consists of parents who are alive and a brother and a sister. The latter is married and lives with her family in Chandigarh. When Amrik came for counselling he was ill with fever and STDs.

Well-built and well dressed, Amrik seemed anxious, fearful and restless during the counselling session. He wanted to go to the cloak room all the time and yet kept drinking water. He was very nervous and insisted on denying the fact that he was HIV-positive. He kept saying *Mere Ko Nahin Ho Sakta* (it can't happen to me) and refused to accept the report. He seemed in a tearing hurry to get the session over with. His answers to questions were filled with contradictions. Married for three years, Amrik had a two-year-old son. The HIV status of his wife and son was not known then.

Amrik had tested HIV-positive at a private laboratory in Mumbai. He was accompanied to the counselling session by his younger brother who was an engineer. He was tested again at the ARCON Centre and was asked to collect his report within a week. But two days after the counselling session, he suddenly developed suspected meningitis and died.

Amrik had an unusual history of inconsistent and anxiety-related avoidance behaviour. According to his elder sister, who had come to Mumbai from Chandigarh on hearing the news of his sudden demise, Amrik had a traumatic childhood. He was teased and bullied at school forcing him to bunk classes. He used to leave home at the right time and return at the allotted hour. But nobody knew where he spent his time because he was not at school. All this happened in the eighth standard.

When his parents got to know about this, he ran away from home. Travelling alone and ticketless by train, he landed up at his paternal aunt's residence in Delhi. When his family found out where he was, he pushed off to another aunt's place. He was finally traced and brought back to Mumbai. This was the start of a lifetime on the run. Amrik's sister felt that his agonising childhood could have been softened by sensitive handling. Instead of being reprimanded all the time, some understanding and empathy would have helped.

As time passed, Amrik's avoidance behaviour pattern replicated in other contexts as well. He kept dropping out of courses until he was inspired to join the Indian Air Force where he appeared to have settled down. But this was short-lived and his erratic behaviour pattern resurfaced.

One day, years ago, Indian Air Force personnel came home inquiring about his whereabouts. Amrik hadn't reported to headquarters after home leave. The mystery deepened because he had also left home. He was finally traced to a friend's home in Delhi. He was jailed by the air force authorities. After a few years, he decided to leave the air force to make more money. He dabbled in various ventures, failed miserably, and returned to his father's transport business.

In Amrik's community, the elder brother's widow is traditionally married off to the younger brother. The family was now under great social pressure to get their daughter-in-law married off to the younger brother, both of whom were of the same age. The brother opposed this move. He didn't want to take care of his sister-in-law and child because, he thought, they would be HIV-positive. He was a computer professional and had planned to find a job and settle down in the United States. But societal pressures had him grounded for the moment. Amrik's wife was keen on the alliance and so were her parents.

Amrik's brother also spoke to the counsellor when Amrik was still alive. He was the sole informant of his brother's HIV status and said that he was under tremendous stress and he wanted to disclose the details to his parents. When he initially came to speak to the counsellor he put up a brave front but broke down soon after a rapport had been built. There was nobody in the family he could talk to. This sharing with the counsellor was like a catharsis for him.

He said he was concerned about Amrik and wanted somebody else to shoulder the responsibility of looking after him before he left for the U.S. He still could not believe how the virus could have infected someone in the family.

Though

his elder sister was a doctor and they knew about HIV/AIDS, he had never ever imagined that the family would have to face the illness at such close quarters. He also wanted to know if his sister-in-law and nephew had to be tested.

He said that his brother had created lots of problems for the family and that his illness was, literally, the last nail in the coffin. He thanked the counsellor for patiently listening to him and told her that he would first talk about the situation to his mother and they would convey it to the father together. The counsellor told him that he could come back whenever he felt the need to talk.

Meanwhile, Amrik's parents hoped that his wife would marry somebody else on the condition that the grandchild would remain with them. They hadn't communicated this to the daughter-in-law directly and expected the counsellor to do it. In fact, for a while, they resisted bringing his wife to the hospital for an HIV test. Several weeks later, she was tested at one of the voluntary testing centres and was found to be reactive.

OBSERVATIONS

* Socio-cultural implications (remarriage of the widow to thebrother-in-law) on the family following HIV-related death is reflected in this case.

* Issue of discrimination and lack of socio-economic and sexual empowerment of a young widow is evident.

* The plight of a widow of an HIV-infected person: the in-laws don't want to keep her and her parents don't want to take her back.

* Diversity of cultural issues among clients should be considered while counselling.

* Psychological consequences of being the sole informant of an incurable illness of a close family member is observed in the client's brother.

* The case brings out the relevance of grief counselling for the family in the event of the death of a close relative.

CASE 8

MARRIED MALE: RESISTANCE TO BEHAVIOUR CHANGE

TWENTY - SEVEN year-old Gautam Kumar was referred to the ARCON Centre for clinical management. He had tested HIV-positive at a private laboratory where he did not receive pre-test counselling. Unaware of the implications of a positive test, he had continued to have unprotected sex with his wife. He came for the counselling session with his four-month old son. He was tested again. His HIV-positive status was confirmed and he was asked to bring his wife for counselling and testing. Gautam keeps coming to the ARCON Centre for the management of his condition but refuses to bring his wife along.

Soft-spoken and well dressed, Gautam has a fairly reasonable job in the eastern suburbs of Mumbai. Despite all the information about HIV at his disposal, there had been no modification in his high-risk behaviour. He had gone ahead and had another child. When he was asked why he refused to use protection, he insisted that there was no point in it as he would have already infected his wife. When he was told about the danger of passing on the virus to his children, he said that he didn't really care and that they would be infected if it was their destiny. It was difficult to reason with him because he simply refused to listen.

Gautam hadn't told his wife about his HIV-positive status. He said he didn't want her to get anxious or tense. The counsellor confronted him and explained that by not engaging in safe sex and by keeping the truth from her, he wasn't giving her any chance to protect herself if she wasn't already infected. If she was infected and didn't know about it, she wouldn't be able to take care of her health or even her children's health in the event of her death. The counsellor gave him the option of bringing his wife to the ARCON Centre so that she could help initiate the process of disclosure. But, till date, Gautam doesn't feel his wife should be told of the situation or even brought for counselling. He, however, comes regularly for medical care.

OBSERVATIONS

* Once again, unethical practice of testing for HIV without counselling is evident.

* Counsellor's role should include helping the client to explore implications of informing the spouse.

* Individual versus shared confidentiality needs to be dealt with during counselling sessions.

* There are apparent contradictions in the client regarding his concern for his wife and children.

* The counsellor's role is significant in exploring the underlying dynamics of contradictions.

* The client has to be helped to take responsibility for his actions and avoiding high risk behaviour.

* The risk of developing STDs in view of unprotected sex needs to be clarified.

* There is need to consider termination of counselling at some stage or consider referral for psychiatric opinion.

CASE 9

WIFE POSITIVE, HUSBAND NEGATIVE: COPING WITH STEREOTYPES

SHEILA RAUT is a twenty-six year-old housewife from a middle-class Maharashtrian family. She was born and brought up in a small town in Maharashtra where she did her schooling and then graduated in Commerce. In college she fell in love with a classmate and had a steady relationship with him for about two years. During this period they had frequent unprotected sexual intercourse until they broke up. Two years later, she had an arranged marriage and moved to Mumbai.

For Shridhar, her husband, it was his second marriage. He also had a two-and-a-half year-old son from the first marriage. To avoid conflict with her in-laws and to contribute to the family kitty, Sheila took up a part-time job in an office nearby. About a year after the marriage she got pregnant. During her routine follow-up, she underwent an HIV test which was reactive. The couple was referred to the ARCON Centre for further tests and counselling.

Sheila came across as a simple woman who appeared to be very attached to her husband. She was five months pregnant at that time and had very little knowledge about HIV/AIDS. She had heard about the disease and that was all. She wasn't particularly worried about her condition. She was more concerned about the chances of infecting her husband. She was open and co-operative and answered all questions with ease. She also revealed to the counsellors the inside story of the husband's first marriage.

Shridhar and his first wife had innumerable marital problems forcing her to ultimately commit suicide. Apparently, the in-laws used to harass her for more dowry. She was a soft and sensitive woman. Since there was no solution in sight to the unending harassment, she had taken her life. That seemed to her the only way out. This had affected Shridhar very badly. He was left with a child to take care of and never stopped blaming himself for not having asserted himself in time. He had no idea that the situation had got out of control and that his wife would commit suicide.

After his marriage to Sheila, Shridhar decided that the couple would be better off staying on their own. He didn't want his parents to interfere this time. But when he heard about Sheila's HIV-positive status, he was distraught. He didn't want to lose her too.

Sheila pointed out that her only sexual partner before marriage was her classmate in college. She had had no blood transfusion and didn't take drugs. It was that love affair which was now threatening to shatter her idyllic existence. It seemed a happy family. Sheila and Shridhar were very much in love and the child was also well adjusted and much sought after by both parents. Like a true self-sacrificing wife, she told the counsellor that she was not worried about herself. It was the health and future of her husband and child that was her foremost concern.

The new dimension to the situation was the child Sheila was carrying. While they wanted to have a child, Sheila and Shridhar also understood the danger of giving birth to a child with a life-threatening disease. After thorough counselling they decided against having the child. When tested again at the ARCON Centre, Sheila tested positive. She was referred to the gynaecology ward of the J.J.Hospital for further management of her pregnancy. To the relief and disbelief of Shridhar, he tested negative. He was advised a repeat test to confirm his negative status.

Sheila was in a quandary. Her family provided full support while her in-laws seemed unsure of what to do. Her life was now at a peculiar crossroads. HIV-positive herself, she believed she would infect the child she was carrying, and her husband may be widowed for the second time.

When Sheila came for the first counselling session, she seemed to send out a silent plea for support and understanding. It was obvious that revealing the sexual episode in college was very difficult. Her apprehensions about being judged was to be carefully handled. Moreover, the need to give priority to her health had to be emphasised. The couple was provided encouragement and support to deal with their unique situation.

OBSERVATIONS

* There was a lack of adequate knowledge of HIV/AIDS despite the couple being literate.

* It possibly reflected on the ineffectiveness of on-going awareness campaigns.

* The husband needed help to cope with the HIV status of the wife.

* There is need for the counsellor to be sensitive to the role of stereotypes like "a self-sacrificing wife" as being detrimental to the client.

* Evidence of fatalism seen in the client.

CASE 10

MARRIED FEMALE: IMPLICATIONS OF UNCONSENTED TESTING

TWENTY-TWO year-old Rajni Pillai tested HIV-positive at a private laboratory and was sent to the ARCON Centre for further tests and counselling. Rajni wasn't told anything about HIV/AIDS, the nature of the test she was asked to take or even the results of the test by her physician. She was carrying her second child and needed more elaborate medical attention. Rajni, however, guessed something was wrong. Her gut feeling told her that something terrible was going to happen. She only hoped and prayed that her child would be safe.

Rajni looked tired and malnourished when she first met the counsellor but was able to grasp what was being said. She asked relevant questions and understood whatever the counsellor told her. Over time, she opened up and relaxed.

During the counselling session she was also provided with general information about food habits, nutrition and a healthy regimen she should adopt. Rajni listened intently to what the counsellor had to say but when it came to the right food habits, she broke down.

She confessed that she would be lucky if she even got a morsel of food at home. She said she usually subsisted on stale food and leftovers. Her mother-in-law and husband ill-treated her. They showed her no respect, love or dignity. She thought even a lowly servant would have been treated better. She had to do all the household chores from dawn to midnight and had to fill water from the common tap till the last days of her pregnancy. She pleaded that the counsellor intervene if she were to get a better deal at home. She told the counsellor to break the news gently to her family without telling them that she had even uttered a word against them.

Rajni came two days later with her husband and mother-in-law. She was being discharged from the hospital and they had come to take her home. The counsellor gave them all the relevant information about HIV/AIDS and how Rajni should be carefully looked after. To this the husband retorted that even he had HIV but he worked hard and didn't complain. The counsellor explained that everybody's needs were different and that Rajni was very weak after the delivery and also had to look after the first child. If she fell ill, the burden of looking after the family would fall on the grandmother.

The counsellor spoke to the mother-in-law privately who painted a rosy picture of a happy and contented family. She said that she had always taken care of her daughter-in-law like her own daughter. The counsellor emphasised that Rajni would require special care. Rajni and her husband were called in to join the discussion. They clarified their doubts and the counsellor gave them all the information required about HIV-related care. The husband realised the gravity of the situation and made a commitment that he would take better care of the entire family.

OBSERVATIONS

* Unethical mandatory HIV testing in the absence of pre-test counselling and consent led to feelings of apprehension and uncertainty.

* Pre-test counselling is useful in psychologically preparing the client to deal with an HIV-positive report.

* The importance of counselling in dealing with secondary transmission of HIV to the partner is highlighted.

* Often, client needs support from the counsellor to deal with family members.

* Role of counsellor in helping the client disclose her HIV status to family members is seen in this case.

* It is important for health care workers to be sensitive to the client's socio-economic status while addressing dietary and other health care needs.

* Counselling for home-based care is essential for clients and family members.

* Discussing the risks and implications of perinatal transmission is necessary for HIV-positive couples.

* Issues of AIDS orphans need to be addressed.

* The responsibility of bringing up the children of HIV-positive parents is likely to fall on the elderly in the family; in this case, the grandmother.

CASE 11

HEARING AND SPEECH IMPAIRED COUPLE: NEW CHALLENGES IN COUNSELLING

MANOJ Thakkar is forty-five years old. He is uneducated, has been married twice and worked as a salesman on a contract basis. Maya, his wife, is fifteen years younger and has been educated till the sixth standard in the Gujarati medium. She works from home, stitching garments for personal clients. They are a hearing and speech impaired couple. They have two children. The older child, a daughter, is able to hear and speak with some difficulty. The son is also hearing and speech impaired.

They are from a lower middle-class background and live in a chawl in Byculla. They earn just enough to run the household and pay the children's school fees. They seem very attached to one another. They have large extended families. Maya has five brothers and three sisters and Manoj has five brothers and five sisters who don't really care for them. This has brought Manoj and Maya even closer. For one another, they are the world.

Well-dressed, smiling a lot and gesticulating widely, they were totally oblivious to the contents of the report of the blood test they were holding in their hands. They seemed happy and content in each other's company. But the cookie had crumbled. Manoj had tested HIV-positive.

This was an unique case. It was a challenge for the counsellor to communicate to the couple through gestures and get her point across. Maya could read simple written Hindi but Manoj was illiterate. Despite the apparent difficulties in communication, the counselling sessions worked well due to the enthusiasm of the couple and the innovativeness of the counsellor.

Manoj had first married around fifteen years ago while he was living in Surat. Apparently, he was forced into marriage. He insisted that he wasn't interested in marrying the woman but circumstances had got the better of him. Maya interrupted at this stage and pointed out that the woman Manoj married even had a bad reputation. Problems erupted immediately after marriage and within two weeks the honeymoon was over.

A few years later, Manoj met Maya. They liked each other and decided to get married. After five years of marriage, they left Surat and moved to Mumbai. They have now been married for ten years and have two children, a daughter in the third standard and a son in the second standard. They communicated that they are happily married and had formed a deep bond between themselves. It seemed cruel in the midst of all this happiness and bonding to burst the bubble and break the news of Manoj's seropositivity, its dangers, implications and consequences.

Both of them had never had a blood transfusion or used

needles and syringes. There was no evidence of any other route of HIV transmission either. After his first marriage, which was fifteen years ago, Manoj admitted to having sex only with Maya. A lot of time had elapsed for the HIV infection to show up. It was only recently that Manoj had begun falling ill on a regular basis. He had had prolonged bouts of unexplained diarrhoea and fever and was advised an HIV test. Maya tested negative and the two children hadn't been tested as yet.

At this juncture and given the unique circumstances of the couple, there was no point in digging up skeletons. There were many grey areas: ten to fifteen years for the HIV infection to show up is rare; also Maya had tested negative. Manoj appeared to be holding something back. Instead of needling him for the finer details, the focus of the counselling sessions was on helping the couple come to grips with the illness which threatened to tear their happiness to pieces.

OBSERVATIONS

* It is a challenge for the counsellor to deal with different groups of people; in this case, the hearing and speech impaired.

* Involvement of the counsellor with the client to an undesirable limit is likely to result in burn-out of the counsellor.

* It is important for the counsellor to avoid forcing the client to disclose any information including the possible transmission routes of his HIV/STD infection.

■ CASE 12 ■

WIDOW: SUPPORT AT WORKPLACE

INDU, a slim, pleasant twenty-four year-old widow, was referred to the ARCON Centre for clinical management. Her husband had died of AIDS a year-and-a-half ago and she had also tested HIV-positive. Indu fully understood her predicament. She was determined to fight her situation.

Indu had no children from the marriage. She had studied till the ninth standard and had fallen in love with Prabir, her late husband, much to the dismay of his parents who had opposed the alliance from the start. Now, they gave her no support whatsoever and she had gone back home to share the tiny family apartment with her father and three younger brothers. Her father was paralysed and her mother was no more. Her three younger brothers had part-time jobs. The family was tolerant but not fully supportive of her situation. The going was tough for everybody.

Indu believes she may have been infected by her husband. She is sure about that. She had no history of blood transfusion. Neither had she taken drugs. Since theirs was a love marriage they knew each other for a long time. But at no time in their relationship did she ever imagine that Prabir would be infected with HIV. He did complain of aches and pains, but that was all. According to her even he wouldn't have known the truth. If he had, she says, he would have told her about it and taken the necessary precautions. She loved him and trusted him and harboured no ill feelings towards him for having passed on the virus.

Indu was very happy and thankful that she had a soul satisfying job. She worked for an NGO project in Kamathipura which helped in the rehabilitation of commercial sex workers and their children. Her work involved information dissemination on HIV/AIDS/STDs.

Indu's area of work needs to be emphasised because she thought it was ironic that while she was telling others to protect themselves from HIV, it was she who had got infected. She couldn't believe it. Despite all the information and knowledge at her disposal, she was here all flesh and blood and seropositive. She was convinced that mere information dissemination wasn't enough. To stem the spread of HIV a lot more needed to be done.

Indu recently moved into a woman's hostel as she didn't want to burden her family with her problems. She explained that her place of work was a source of great support. Her colleagues were wonderful and were always there for her. She admits to getting depressed sometimes and thinks of her husband. Did he know the truth and keep it deliberately from her? But then she hastily wipes these thoughts away. She has realised that keeping busy helps. The past is dead and gone and she has to take control of her present.

Indu has also realised the chasm between theory and practice. She used to tell HIV-positive women that they should take charge of their lives but she now knows how difficult it is. Especially for those who are economically and emotionally dependent on their families. She also felt that the AIDS intervention campaigns had many dangerous gaps that needed to be urgently filled. Her life, she said, would be spent making that happen.

The counselling sessions consisted of sharing information because Indu was also a care provider. As her constructive coping mechanism was identified in the earlier sessions, the later sessions emphasised goal setting for treatment, shelter and other support needs. She was also encouraged to build support from within by identifying her strengths and motivating her to use them to face the future.

OBSERVATIONS

* The ineffectiveness of ongoing health information campaigns.

* The tendency to perceive HIV/AIDS as someone else's disease.

* Evidence of determination in the client to fight the situation. It was used by the counsellor to help strengthen the client's coping mechanism.

* Positive effects of social support were observed in the client.

* The emphasis during counselling was on using the present as a means of constructive coping.

* The case highlights the fact that resources are needed to establish support groups which can assist others in a similar predicament.

■ CASE 13 ■

WIDOW WITH HIV-POSITIVE CHILD: REMARRIED AND PREGNANT

THIRTY year-old Urmila is a tall, fair, thin, soft-spoken middle-class woman. She has completed her secondary school in the Marathi medium. Originally from Satara, her family consists of parents, one brother and two sisters. All her siblings are married.

In 1990 she married a businessman from Parel who died one-and-a-half years later in a car accident near his native place in Sangli. It was an arranged marriage. Within a month of the marriage Urmila was pregnant. Her husband expired when Shaila, the daughter, was five-and-a-half months old.

In 1993 Urmila entered into another arranged marriage to a salesman from the Kalbadevi cloth market. She now stays with her husband and his parents and her daughter Shaila in Borivili, a distant Mumbai suburb.

Urmila had unprotected sex with her second husband for almost a year. She developed genital lesions for which she went to a private clinic in Borivili and was advised an HIV test. When she tested HIV-positive, she was referred to the ARCON Centre along with her second husband and daughter.

The first husband had no history of blood transfusion or of taking drugs and had no known sexual exposure outside marriage. He was known to smoke and drink only on social occasions. There was very little knowledge about his sexual history and HIV status before marriage.

In the first counselling session, Urmila was clad in a pastel coloured cotton sari. She was very shy and self-conscious in her husband's presence and allowed him to do most of the talking. She was content to listen.

Mahesh, the second husband, was a tall, very thin and friendly man. He was very concerned about Shaila. He made it a point to inform the counsellor that if anything happened to her the family would be devastated.

Thirty years old, Mahesh had also studied till the secondary section in the Marathi medium. He was a resident of Virar. He married Urmila in 1993; his first marriage. His family consisted of parents and three sisters, all of whom were married. He tested HIV-positive two years after marriage. He is asymptomatic. Mahesh had a history of unprotected sex with commercial sex workers. Therefore, prior infection cannot be ruled out. He had unprotected sex with his wife before she tested positive. Since then he has always taken precautions.

Mahesh was very concerned about Shaila and loved her as a father should, but still felt incomplete without a child of his own. His parents and sisters were aware of the HIV status of the couple and were very supportive. But they also felt he should have a child!

Shaila is a thin, short and dark girl who is six-and-a-half years old. She had tested HIV-positive two years ago. At that time, she was asymptomatic. Since she has had no history of blood transfusion, the likely route of HIV transmission is from her mother.

Her illness has taken a visible toll. Shaila is underdeveloped for her age. She comes for regular follow-up sessions and has also been put on an ayurvedic drug regimen. However, after recurrent opportunistic infections from April 1998, she has stopped going to school. She was admitted to the paediatrics ward of the J.J.Hospital in Mumbai in a serious condition where she was put on a two-drug anti-retroviral therapy. She is now a case of AIDS.

Shaila is also very intelligent but her illness has made her very subdued. However, when she attends the counselling sessions, she is animated and talks non-stop. She talks about her school, friends, grandparents and everything else that excites her. She regrets not being able to attend school regularly due to her illness. She is cut off from her peers and is unable to develop the bonds schoolchildren build. But she feels compensated because she is deeply loved by her parents and is always provided with expensive clothes. She admits to being pampered by her paternal grandfather who fulfils all her wishes.

The counsellor explained to the parents the implications of having a second child. The parents admitted that they were fully aware of the consequences and were willing to take the chance. If they succumbed to AIDS, the in-laws had agreed to take care of the child. Urmila is very concerned about

Shaila's welfare but is also keen to have a second child to please her husband and in-laws. Along with that desire is also the worry that the second child may test HIV-positive!

OBSERVATIONS

* Use of specific counselling techniques for children who test HIV-positive. For example, techniques of behaviour modification and play therapy are important tools.

* Mahesh's need to have his own offspring despite knowing his HIV status needs to be considered.

* Need for family counselling was identified considering the pressures on the couple to have a child.

* Evidence of family support following disclosure of HIV status by the client to family members.

* Urmila's dilemma of social pressures on one hand and the implications of her HIV status on the pregnancy on the other needs to be addressed.

* Counsellor's role is only to present options to the client. Decision making is the sole prerogative of the client.

CASE 14

WIDOWER: FAMILY RESPONSIBILITY AND GOAL SETTING FOR HIS CHILDREN

YASHWANT Rana is forty-five years old. He has studied till the higher secondary stage in the Hindi medium and works as a lift operator in a tyre company. He is a widower. His wife succumbed to AIDS four years ago leaving behind two sons and three daughters, the youngest of whom is still at school. Yashwant is not only HIV-positive but is also the only earning member of the family burdened with the responsibility of having to take care of his growing children.

Yashwant is a very simple looking man dressed in an ordinary white kurta-pyjama. He wears a gold stud on his left earlobe and speaks Hindi with a distinct Uttar Pradesh accent. He has kept his HIV status hidden from everybody, especially his children, in a bid to shield them from any type of social ostracism. He has no support systems and has to fight the battle on his own. His brothers and mother who live back home in Uttar Pradesh are involved in their own affairs and know nothing of what is happening in Yashwant's life.

Yashwant feels that he has been infected by his wife, the late Durga Bai, as he has never had any sexual exposure outside marriage or a blood transfusion or a history of IV drug abuse. In most cases, the husband infects the wife. Here, it seems, it is the other way around. When Durga was pregnant with their sixth child, complications arose during delivery which necessitated a blood transfusion. Events then took a sad turn. Durga lost the child, contracted HIV from the blood transfused and later passed on the virus to Yashwant. Durga took ill and died. Yashwant tested HIV-positive soon after and his entire life went into a tailspin.

Yashwant kept the details of his wife's death and his seropositive status a closely guarded secret. He was wary of societal reactions. He was also under tremendous pressure. The younger children would never understand AIDS and the older daughter's chances of getting married would be permanently marred. All this stress was getting the better of him. A stocky, well-built man, he was now exhibiting symptoms of growing weakness. He confessed that the pressure was getting increasingly difficult to handle.

As Yashwant's immune system was getting debilitated by the day, he began feeling sick more often and felt like lying down most of the time. Seeing him in a comatose state his younger children would constantly inquire why he wasn't going to work. Initially, he gave them silly excuses but now, as his health deteriorates further, his reasons are wearing thin.

The counselling sessions provided Yashwant an opportunity to talk. It allowed him to express his feelings which were bottled up deep within. In the process of counselling, he was encouraged to consider the pros and cons of disclosing his HIV-positive status to others. Over subsequent follow-up sessions, the counsellor explored whether the consequences of disclosure would be detrimental to the client.

It was important to consider the fact that as illness progressed, increasing symptoms might show up and the children might have more embarrassing questions. On the other hand, the advantages of revealing his HIV-positive status could include more support and less conflict from his family. Constructive planning and goal setting for his children was another aspect touched upon during counselling.

Yashwant pointed out that he had come to terms with his illness. His only concern was the well-being of his children should something happen to him. He had found solace in God and spirituality. It helped him maintain a semblance of sanity and had also kept him motivated. He planned to educate his children and marry off his daughters. After that, he said, he was ready to die. Yashwant has accepted his condition. He has a positive attitude which has brought him this far and will probably carry him through.

OBSERVATIONS

* Fear of social stigma and discrimination was evident in the client because of his HIV-positive status.

* The counsellor needs to encourage the development of coping mechanisms of the client for dealing with the psychological consequences of HIV.

* The role of disclosure in eliciting social support has to be elucidated in the counselling process.

* Acceptance of death as an inevitability for all mortals needs to be incorporated in HIV/AIDS counselling.

* Goal setting is an important motivating factor for positive living.

* Role of spirituality has to be explored in dealing with crises.

CASE 15

MALE DIVORCEE: LONELINESS AND LACK OF SUPPORT FOR THE ELDERLY

SHAMMI Singh is a sixty-two year-old divorcee who has a son who lives in the United States and a daughter who is married and stays in Pune. His son stayed back in the United States after going there on a tourist visa many years ago and his daughter and her husband, who he is not particularly fond of, run a real-estate business. He has been divorced for over ten years and lives all alone in a posh south Mumbai residential area.

From an upper class background, Shammi was in the garment business. His ex-wife has remarried and they are not in touch. His children also lead their own lives and have no contact with the father. Shammi has been left on his own for a long time and has no support systems.

In 1963 Shammi had undergone a hernia operation. He was required to undergo another hernia operation recently for which a blood test was done and Shammi turned out to be HIV-positive. He abandoned the operation and began scanning all information related to HIV/AIDS. He had heard about the ARCON Centre and decided to drop in.

Considering Shammi's socio-economic background, his appearance was one of gross neglect. He wore a white shirt and grey trousers which were crumpled and unwashed. He hadn't shaved for days, there was a thick stubble on his cheeks, his hair was untidy and he wore an unkempt look. His shoulders were stooped. He looked depressed, anxious and defeated. He tried to appear as nonchalant as possible but that was only a mask with gaping holes in it.

A self-confessed loner, Shammi lived in a little island of his own making. He never reached out to others and had very few meaningful relationships. He had no contact with his siblings or children and his parents had expired when he was very young. He said that he was not a great father from the very beginning. Preoccupied with work, he had no time for his children. He didn't have a stable career graph either.

Shammi also moved rapidly from one affair to another. When he was working in Rajasthan as a young man he had an affair with the wife of his landlord. The landlord discovered the relationship and threw his wife out of the house. The lady presented herself at Shammi's doorstep as she had nowhere to go. They began living together. It was a satisfying relationship with no great expectations from either side. He then shifted to Mumbai where he got married. He tried to maintain both the women but his wife started getting suspicious. Sordid marital squabbles led to a divorce after nineteen years of marriage.

Shammi then got involved in a spate of affairs. He also had a number of one-night stands and consorted regularly with call girls and even experimented with recreational drugs.

He had the money and was unattached. So he felt no qualms about it. All along there was no relationship in which he had invested emotions. He had no close friend or somebody he could confide in.

After testing HIV-positive, Shammi admitted to feeling alone and without any support to turn to. He was interested in finding out various treatment modalities. His greatest worry though was how he would manage if he was sick and bedridden. He wanted to know if there was any institution that would take care of him in his last days.

Shammi appeared calm and collected when he came for counselling. However, from his appearance and non-verbal gestures, it appeared as if he had some level of anxiety. The counsellor helped Shammi examine his feelings of loneliness and uncertainty.The importance of establishing and maintaining a social support network was explained. He was encouraged to come for follow-up sessions and to join the support groups for People Living With HIV/AIDS (PLWHA).

OBSERVATIONS

* It is necessary to pay attention to the non-verbal cues of the client.

* The ultimate goal of the counsellor is to help the client get aware of and deal with varied emotions like depression, anxiety, loneliness or defeat.

* In the presence of the client's denial, it is important for the counsellor to explore the psychological framework of the client.

* Role of social skills training is relevant in this case.

* Relevance of hospice care is highlighted.

* Referral to self-help groups can be an option for support.

■ CASE 16 ■

AIDS ORPHANS: ISSUES OF CARE AND SUPPORT

SIX-YEAR-old Nita, a precocious child is HIV-positive and an orphan. Lively, energetic and talkative, she had no inhibitions of talking to the counsellor or of even being in unfamiliar hospital surroundings. She was accompanied to the ARCON Centre by a nurse working with an NGO in suburban Mumbai which took care of other orphaned children like Nita. She came bounding in, holding on to the fingers of the *tai* (as the nurse was called by the children of the orphanage). Every now and then she bounced and skipped a few steps ahead of the *tai*.

When asked to by the counsellor, Nita readily hopped on to a chair. With very little prompting, she told the counsellor that her favourite colour was red and that she liked Hindi film songs. She listed the names of her friends, recited a poem, and when given a blank sheet of paper, enthusiastically sketched on it . She then spontaneously asked the counsellor her name and if she could take the pictures she had sketched "home" (referring to the orphanage).

The nurse explained that Nita was brought to the orphanage when she was three months old by her mother who was destitute, HIV-positive and sick. The whereabouts of her father were unknown. The orphanage took the child in. Soon after, Nita's mother took seriously ill and was hospitalised. She expired within fifteen days. Three years ago, when she was two, Nita tested HIV-positive.

The orphanage has been Nita's home ever since she was brought there as a baby. There are eighteen other children between the ages of two and ten. Five *bais* and two nurses attend to their needs through the day and night.

Generally, most children get adopted by families when they are still babies. Many of the adoptive parents are foreigners. But in Nita's case, considering her illness, adoption seems an highly unlikely option.

The NGO has taken the responsibility of looking after her medical needs. They also pay for her medicines. But when Nita's laboratory reports were compared over a period of six months, no improvement was observed. This gave rise to a number of crucial questions. Was the right dose of medicines being administered to her? Were her caretakers monitoring her condition as carefully as they should?

Despite all this, Nita's spirits were miraculously untouched. She seemed to be oblivious of her unique circumstances. She is an orphan and is HIV-positive. What the future holds for her is anybody's guess.

OBSERVATIONS

* Acceptability of HIV-positive orphans in orphanages is an issue that needs immediate attention.

* An important emerging question is whether orphanages will become hospices for HIV-infected children.

* Society has a responsibility towards the rehabilitation and care of AIDS orphans. This is likely to emerge as a major challenge in India.

* Disclosure of HIV infection to a child is a delicate issue that needs to be thought over and discussed further.

* Caretaker compliance in terms of dose and duration of treatment is vital.

CASE 17

LIVE-IN RELATIONSHIP: CHALLENGES IN THE AIDS ERA

SAIRA and George came together for the counselling session. They made a compatible couple. She was tall, fair and sophisticated. Dressed in blue denims and a white T-shirt, she asked relevant questions in impeccable English. She was outspoken, assertive and wanted to know everything about AIDS: its symptoms, its management, the lifespan of an affected individual, medication required and so on.

George was a tall, well dressed and charming man. He said he knew all about AIDS as he surfed the net regularly. He didn't talk much. Instead, he spent the time listening intently to the conversation between Saira and the counsellor. He felt Saira was too unconcerned about the risk of being infected and felt she required counselling. It was he who insisted she meet the counsellor.

Saira's story:

"My name is Saira. I am thirty years old. I am a post graduate in fashion designing. I come from a very orthodox Muslim family. My parents didn't want me to take up fashion designing as a career, but I was always a rebel. I have been living independently in my own apartment for the last five years. My parents are so strict that I felt suffocated living with them. They objected to everything I did. Imagine, they wanted me to get married at eighteen!

"Last year I met George who is thirty-one years old and works as an advertising executive. I found him very attractive; the proverbial tall, dark and handsome type. He has a great sense of humour, is very considerate and is also very honest, a quality which I treasure.

"We began dating regularly and after six months I decided to move in with him. We began living together in his apartment. It was then that George told me about his HIV-positive status. He was very honest to admit that he had casual sex with multiple partners. He confessed to have led a very fast life but after meeting me he had stopped all this.

"I loved George even more for his honesty. I told him that his HIV-positive status didn't bother me. We had unprotected sex a few times after which George became very restless. He insisted on using a condom and also wanted me to get an ELISA test done. He also felt I needed counselling. I agreed for his sake. Anyway, my blood test was negative. Prior to meeting George I had no exposure to the virus. I didn't do drugs, never had a blood transfusion or sexual exposure.

"The counsellor said that a repeat test after three months would confirm my HIV status. She also told me that George was presently asymptomatic. The asymptomatic period could stretch for a number of years. However, every time we had unprotected sex, he could pass the virus to me. The counsellor also explained how HIV damages the immune system.

"The counsellor and I discussed the importance of emotional and social support and this helped me to understand how re-establishing contact with my family would help. I always thought, in a hopelessly romantic way, that George and I would die together. But after my discussion with the counsellor I realised this might not happen.

"I promised myself that I would never again indulge in unprotected sex and that I would make sincere attempts to regain my parents' love and support. I have realised that I cannot deny reality. I have to face it frontally. The best and the only way is to face it with courage."

OBSERVATIONS

* Varied socio-economic strata from which cases emerge is evident.

* Understanding the need and importance of social support for the client is beneficial.

* There is a great necessity for the counsellor to be abreast of the latest information on HIV/AIDS.

* The different dynamics underlying Saira's decision to live with George could be love, total acceptance, intense emotional dependence or denial of the risk of infection.

* Highlighting various options available to the client is crucial.

* A realistic view of the situation has to be developed.

* The counsellor needs to help the client to make decisions for behaviour change.

CASE 18

SINGLE FEMALE: DEVELOPING ASSERTIVE SKILLS

NILOFER, a twenty-one year-old final year college student, was referred to the ARCON Centre for HIV testing. She had unprotected sex with her boyfriend a couple of months ago and was worried sick she would test HIV-positive.

Pleasant looking and well dressed, Nilofer was also training to be a beautician. Her family consisted of a mother and three sisters. Nilofer stayed with her mother and a married sister in the central suburbs of Mumbai.

Nilofer met Arjun at a friend's place many months ago. They started dating regularly without telling anybody about it. There was great chemistry between them which soon developed into intense fondness. They also grew physically intimate but Nilofer refused to go the whole way. She wanted to, she said, but was petrified. She said she loved Arjun and wanted to share various aspects of his life but was also very confused about her feelings for him.

One day, Arjun booked a room in a hotel and they made love. Nilofer was unable to recollect whether they had penetrative sex. But she was in great distress after this. She discussed the incident with her elder sister and brother-in-law who asked her to go in for an HIV test.

At the pre-test counselling session, Nilofer told the counsellor she was madly in love with Arjun and would do anything for him. He was kind and understanding and had never forced himself on her. She just didn't want to displease him. Of course, she also wanted him as much as he wanted her.

The counsellor probed further about what Nilofer felt about the relationship. She admitted that she was not quite sure about Arjun's feelings for her. The fact that their relationship was a big secret made it worse. She said she had no reason to believe Arjun was HIV-positive or for that matter no reason to believe he wasn't either. She hadn't told him that she had gone for an HIV test. All this non-communication only made it worse. Nilofer also wasn't sure about Arjun's commitment towards the relationship.

The counsellor explained to Nilofer that she would be comfortable in a physical relationship when she was mentally and emotionally sure of the other person. She needn't give in because she felt obliged to or was being emotionally blackmailed. Apart from HIV, a woman may also want to be careful about unwanted pregnancy. The counsellor emphasised that Nilofer and Arjun could communicate at a deeper level. That would help develop mutual trust and respect.

Nilofer tested negative. She was asked to repeat the test after three months and the concept of the window period was explained to her. Since she appeared very worried, the P.C.R. (Polymerase Chain Reaction), which is capable of detecting the HIV infection within two weeks, was also explained to her.

OBSERVATIONS

* Apparent contradictions about the relationship between the client and her boyfriend were communicated by the client.

* Insight in the client can be developed using the confrontation technique to help her see the relationship in the proper perspective.

* Focus of the follow-up counselling sessions could be towards training the client in communication skills and assertiveness.

* Client could be educated about STDs using pictorial charts.

CASE 19

MARRIED MALE: RESISTANCE TO COUNSELLING

REHAMAT Khan is twenty-nine years old. He has studied till the eighth standard and worked as an unskilled labourer in a factory mixing chemicals for the manufacture of dyes.

Well-dressed, calm and composed, he betrayed no trace of anxiety. He had tested HIV-positive and had been sent to the ARCON Centre for counselling. He listened to all that the counsellor had to say without interrupting even once and spoke only when asked to. He seemed completely indifferent to the situation. Rehamat wore a bland, almost bored expression although he had tested HIV-positive only the day before. He was either in complete denial or had such a laidback personality that nothing seemed to affect him.

Rehamat was married about six years ago and had two children, a daughter aged five and a son aged three. He gave a history of outside sexual exposure two years after marriage. He had heard about AIDS but believed it could never happen to him and that it was somebody else's disease.

When Rehamat came to the ARCON Centre he complained of substantial weight loss and continuous fever for about two months. When asked about his lifestyle he answered in monosyllables. He didn't volunteer information. When asked about his thoughts and feelings, he said he was not anxious. He said he had no tension. As long as he could eat and drink, everything was fine by him.

It was important to know if Rehamat had grasped the seriousness of the situation. Without frightening him, it was necessary to tell him the implications of his diagnosis. He could then take precautions to avoid infecting his wife who had not yet been tested, and also take medication for any opportunistic infections that would arise. It was important to tell him about safe sex, the necessity to boost his immune system and the need to reduce stress levels. He had admitted to a fondness for country liquor. That would have to be avoided. Aspects of confidentiality, the discrimination he was likely to face and future planning should something happen to him would also have to be considered.

OBSERVATIONS

* Reactions to a positive HIV test report could be varied.

* Apparent indifference on the part of the client could be interpreted as total denial or as a lack of understanding of the implications of testing HIV-positive.

* Professional challenges in counselling includes dealing with clients who have varied personality dispositions.

* Counselling to be directed towards helping the client undertake future planning and goal setting.

CASE 20

HEALTH CARE PROVIDERS: PROFESSIONAL DILEMMAS

TWENTY-THREE year-old Shyamsunder was referred to the ARCON Centre for a blood test to determine his CD4/CD8 count. Unmarried and working as an assistant laboratory technician at a regional hospital, he was the youngest of three children. His family was well educated. Both his elder sisters were post-graduates and had well paid jobs. His father was a social worker and his mother a teacher.

Shyamsunder had a needle prick injury a year ago when he had just finished taking the blood sample of a patient whose HIV status was not known. The needle had pricked his forefinger when he was trying to cap it. At that time, the senior laboratory technician present told him not to worry about it and to simply wash the affected part with antiseptic. Shyamsunder did just that and forgot about it. Later, when he came to know that the patient whose blood sample he had taken was HIV-positive, he got himself tested. Shyamsunder turned out to be positive too. The dramatic turn of events was a shock for everyone concerned.

He was referred to a doctor in Mumbai who in turn directed him to the ARCON Centre. His father, uncle and the doctor accompanied him for the pre-test counselling.

Of average build, well dressed and calm, Shyamsunder was very cooperative with the counsellors. He spoke openly about his emotions now that he had tested HIV-positive. He didn't present any history of blood transfusion or sexual exposure.

Shyamsunder was very close to his family and felt he had let them down. He said he would now be unable to fulfil the expectations of an only son. He had hoped to save enough money to keep his parents in comfort after retirement. He also wanted to marry off his sisters in great style. Now he wouldn't be able to do all this. He also wanted to get married and enjoy the pleasures of being a father. All his dreams had come crashing down.

Shyamsunder kept talking, his words pouring out like torrential rain. His greatest anxiety now, he confessed, was disclosing his HIV status to his mother. It would break her heart and he just didn't want to hurt her in any way. He wanted to tell her the truth himself and had requested his father not to break the news. As an afterthought he confessed that he wouldn't be telling his mother about it right away. In fact, he may never tell her about it. It would only complicate matters. He would wait till his sisters were married and settled and then maybe wait till his mother brought up the issue of his marriage.

As a laboratory technician, Shyamsunder was fully aware of AIDS and its ramifications. He needed no education on the technical aspects of his predicament. But he desperately needed a shoulder to lean on. Over a period of time, Shyamsunder developed a good rapport with the counsellor and was ready to face whatever life had to offer.

The counsellor convinced him that there was no need to feel guilty for what had happened and to move ahead. It was not the end of the world. With careful planning he felt he would be able to cope.

His mood improved. He became more cheerful and began looking at life with hope. The only worry which still remained as far as he was concerned was how he would convey the news to his mother. The counsellor told him not to rush into it and take his father's help. With time, the coping mechanisms would be strengthened.

The counsellor asked him to chalk out his priorities. His foremost priority was adjusting to his HIV-positive status and then telling his mother about it. The counsellor told him that since he had decided on his priorities, he should work on them one at a time. Shyamsunder decided to take rational decisions and not allow his problem to overcome him.

OBSERVATIONS

* Variety of emotions such as anxiety, loss of self-worth and failure to meet expectations were observed in the client.

* Counsellor's role in helping the client to deal with emotions is evident in this case.

* Multiple needle pricks is a professional hazard and health care workers need to be updated on the precautions necessary.

* The need to take care while using needles and sharp instruments is to be emphasised.

* Reported occupational risk of HIV transmission in health care workers is 0.03%.

CASE 21

FALSE HIV REPORT: PSYCHOLOGICAL TRAUMA

RAM Sharma, a forty-two year-old married man, was referred to the ARCON Centre for an HIV test. He had an HIV report from a private laboratory which said he was HIV non-reactive. Ram wasn't satisfied with the report and so got another ELISA test done from another laboratory which also said he was HIV non-reactive. To confirm the report he got a P.C.R. done at yet another laboratory which said he was positive for HIV-1.

Greatly distressed by the last report, Ram had come to the ARCON Centre for further testing and, if necessary, clinical management. Since all new cases are tested afresh, the usual procedures were followed. After the necessary pre-test counselling, Ram's blood sample was taken. The report said Ram had no HIV antibodies. Ram was still dissatisfied and insisted on another HIV test.

Intrigued by his insistence, the counsellor explored Ram's background to fully understand his paranoia.

Ram had been married for the last twenty years. He had two children and a stable income from a government job. He was well-built and apparently healthy. He was also always well dressed and very cooperative with the counsellor. His comprehension level was high and he asked questions and provided answers when required.

He had no history of blood transfusions. His last sexual exposure with his spouse, he said, was four years ago and it was non-penetrative. He had one incident of sexual exposure outside marriage. It was a passive homosexual exposure at a public urinal where, he claimed, he was seduced. He had oral sex on that occasion. Barring this incident, Ram insisted that he had no other sexual exposure.

Ever since, Ram was torn by guilt. He confessed that the doctors at the ARCON Centre and the counsellor were the only ones he had shared this experience with. He felt ashamed for what he had done and felt he deserved to get HIV for the immoral act he had engaged in. The fact that he got a false P.C.R. report egged his imagination and fears even further. He got another P.C.R. report which also said he was non-reactive. But Ram was still dissatisfied. He was convinced he was going to suffer for the rest of his life. He was also worried he would infect his children.

The counsellor repeatedly told Ram that the reports showed that he didn't have HIV and would in no way infect his children. But Ram remained resolutely unconvinced. During further follow-up sessions, the counsellor asked the client to present the rationale for accepting the positive report and not the negative ones. This led the client to understand that the isolated positive report could be an aberration. He slowly settled down to the fact that he wasn't HIV-positive and wouldn't need to test his children for HIV either.

OBSERVATIONS

* Test results of clients need to be interpreted in conjunction with case history.

* Care needs to be taken in handling samples to be tested for HIV.

* It is necessary to understand the psychological framework of the client before initiating any intervention.

* Client's reactions to HIV are influenced by his cultural, moral and ethical framework.

* There is a necessity of repeatedly clarifying myths and misconceptions regarding HIV/AIDS.

* Importance of confrontation as a technique in the development of insight/acceptance of the client is reflected in this case.

* It is essential that the health care worker informs the client of the likely false result that could be obtained on a single ELISA test.

WOMEN AND AIDS

Here I am, a few years on
It was hard enough explaining where Daddy had gone
She knows there's something far wrong with me
How can I explain about HIV
I see the sadness, the fear in her eyes
Each time I have to be hospitalised
and I see the way she looks at me
Each time I take my AZT
'I thought these pills were to make you well,
So why are you still sick then, go on mum tell
Quick mum, here, be sick in this basin'
I can see within her tiny mind racing
'I'll help you mum watch you don't fall'
and she treats me like a china doll
Then the moments for something, I was very scared
The question that I had not prepared
'Why do I get a jag mum, why do I get blood taken?'
The moment of truth now there can be no faken
'Well it's the doctor's special way of knowing
that inside you there's no bugs growing
Tiny bugs that can make you unwell'
I had no choice but the truth to tell
'You don't have these bugs darling, so there's no need to worry'
'But you have, mummy,' she says in a hurry
'Yes my lamb, in me these bugs grow'
'When you die mummy, where will I go?'

I don't know the answer to that question
Instead I made this stupid suggestion
Shall we go to the fridge and get some Ice Cream
Then we had a cuddle, and I said I'm here
I wish I could take away all her fear
her blood just now may not be infected
but by HIV she is most definitely affected
I don't fear dying anymore
Just for a special little girl who's only four.

Courtesy: Working with Women & AIDS.

Compiled by Jyoti Bakshani.

AIDS RESEARCH AND CONTROL (ARCON) CENTRE

ARCON Centre is a technical organisation established under the collaborative programme of the Government of Maharashtra and the University of Texas-Houston, USA. The primary objectives of ARCON are to promote interaction and collaboration in the areas of research and training and to develop academic, scientific, clinical and cultural relationships by providing faculty and students with educational research experience. ARCON is managed by senior officials of the Government of Maharashtra and the University of Texas.

ARCON has the following specific mandates :

1. To conduct medical and behavioural research.
2. Training of health care workers.
3. Develop replicable models for priority interventions.
4. Provide technical expertise to the state of Maharashtra, the Government of India and international agencies.

RESEARCH

ARCON, primarily being a technical organisation, has special emphasis on research. Over 30 research projects, both medical and behavioural, have been commissioned. Important among them are the natural history of HIV among adult and children, transmission studies (heterosexual and mother to baby), interaction between HIV and tuberculosis, interactions between HIV and conventional Sexually

Transmitted Infections (STI), clinical spectrum in adults and children, spectrum of opportunistic infections with AIDS, effectiveness of combination anti-retroviral and ayurvedic drugs, models of care in hospitals and communities, and mortality studies. Findings of these studies provide useful data for developing national strategies. Behavioural research projects involve studying the impact of counselling and developing strategies to sustain sexual behaviour change of individuals over a period of time.

ARCON has published 27 scientific papers in national and international journals, contributed chapters in local and international textbooks, and participated in over 30 international conferences.

TECHNICAL EXPERTISE

ARCON works with governments, non-governmental agencies and the private sector in developing systems to replicate successful experiences related to HIV/AIDS.

ARCON provides technical assistance to the National AIDS Control Organisation (NACO) of the Government of India, various state governments, and UN and international agencies in implementing preventive and supportive programmes to strengthen the national response to HIV/AIDS.